HCG Diet Recipes and Cookbook

50 HCG Diet Recipes + Our Free HCG Diet Summary - Get the Secret HCG Recipes that Everyone is Looking for...

Written By: M. Smith & R. King
Edited by: Country Cooking Publishing

HCG Diet Recipes and Cookbook

Edited by: Country Cooking Publishing

"You must begin to think of yourself as becoming the person you want to be". **David Viscott**

Table of Contents

The HCG Diet Summary

The HCG Diet

Many may have heard of the diet where you can lose 1 to 3 pounds a day, stay active and maintain the weight loss for the rest of your life. This diet is known as the hcg diet. HCG is human chronic gonadotropin. This natural protein hormone is developed during the first trimester of pregnancy and is a class of hormone that is concealed in the blood stream. These hormones aide in the function of the endocrine, pituitary and hypothalamus glands which are found in the human body. This hormone is believed to send signals to the body that helps in breaking down and using body fat to fuel the body.

When on a low calorie diet the muscle mass in the body begins to deplete. This in turn lowers the resting metabolism rate of the body. For every 1 lb of muscle you lose you also lose about 50 calories. Meaning that if you lose muscle you are losing metabolism or the amount of energy the body burns to maintain. HCG stops the body from following this train of thought. It basically tricks the body into believing it is getting the calories so it remains full of energy and keeps you active.

It is true that if you maintain a low calorie diet you will lose weight. The bad part of a low calorie diet is that you may lose weight but you are not losing fat. It's muscle that you lose. This is why your metabolism slows down when on a low calorie diet. HCG helps to keep the metabolism in check and helps in achieving lasting results from the diet.

The HCG diet includes three phases to help you achieve your goals.

PHASE 1

This phase lasts for 21 consecutive days. It consists of taking the hcg serum. It also includes a 500 calorie a day diet of specific foods with specific amounts. On the first two days you can pretty much eat whatever you like. On the third day it's the 500 calorie a day plan. These foods include proteins that will help maintain an active lifestyle. Eating a 500 calorie a day diet can leave you feeling tired and out of energy but with this diet you can stay active and still lose the weight you want. In fact it is said on the hcg diet you can lose 1 to 3 pounds a day.

PHASE 2

This phase also has duration of 21 days. It includes a specific herb mix that is said to help recreate set points in 3 major glands. These glands include the pituitary gland, the endocrine gland and the hypothalamus gland. Maintaining these set points is critical to losing fat.

Most of us know what the pituitary and endocrine gland are. The pituitary gland is at the base of the brain and it secrets hormones to the body. The endocrine gland is the main gland in the endocrine system that releases hormones through the blood stream.

The hypothalamus gland is also a very small gland in the brain. It not only regulates hormones but also body temperature and metabolism. It is crucial to regulate these glands when on a low calorie diet. The hcg diet helps in doing that.

PHASE 3

This phase is called “Clean and healthy eating for life,” It helps to maintain your weight loss thru diet for the rest of your life. Stick to the exact diet for maintaining the body weight you have achieved over phase 1 and 2.

It may be hard to find the right foods to eat in the right amounts when it comes to the hcg diet. For the most part chicken, fish, seafood and beef can be eaten in small amounts, usually about 3.5 oz. Fresh or frozen fruits and vegetables are also a part of the diet. It’s best to start out with only 1 serving a day and try to keep it to 3.5 oz. You can adjust to 2 servings in phase 2 and 3 of the diet.

Nuts and seeds are also on the list. Start with 1 serving a day and keep it at 1 oz. It’s best to eat nuts and seeds in the raw state. This will ensure that no enzymes are lost through heating and cooking. To find the exact foods and amounts do your research. There are numerous Internet sites that can help you in finding the right foods to eat on the hcg diet.

Although the hcg diet consists of specific foods in specific amounts you still need to stay away from the fatty foods. If you follow the diet protocol and eat only the recommended foods weight loss will be a breeze. As always talk with your doctor before making a drastic change such as this diet.

HCG Diet Recipes

Spiced Breakfast Bake

Spiced Breakfast Bake

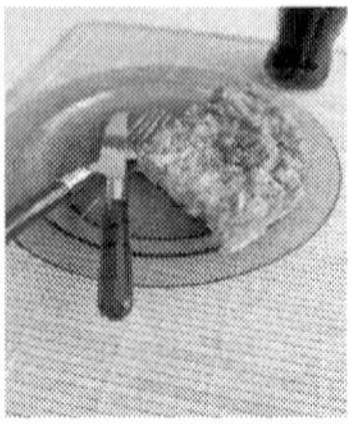

Ingredients:

4 eggs

4 egg whites

1/4 tsp cayenne pepper

1/2 green bell pepper, diced

1/2 sweet red pepper, diced

1 small onion, diced

6 pieces of turkey bacon, diced

1 (10 oz.) can tomato and green chilies, drained well

1/2 Pepper Jack cheese, shredded

Directions:

Place the whole eggs and the egg whites into a bowl.

Add the cayenne pepper and whisk until blended well.

Place the peppers, onion and bacon into a skillet.

Place the skillet over medium high heat and sauté 5 minutes or until tender.

Pour the egg mixture into a pie plate.

Stir in the bacon mixture, tomatoes and cheese.

Bake the casserole in a preheated 375 degree oven for 40 minutes or until the eggs are cooked through.

Seafood Omelet

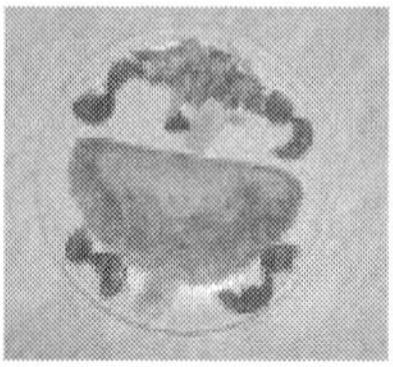

Ingredients:

Coconut oil

2 oz. of egg beaters

1/4 tsp thyme

1/8 tsp basil

1/8 tsp liquid Stevia

1 oz. crab meat

1 oz. shrimp, diced

1/8 tsp sea salt

Directions:

Lightly grease a frying pan with a little coconut oil.

Mix the egg beaters, thyme, basil and sweetener together in a mixing bowl.

Heat the pan over medium heat and add the egg beater mixture.

In a bowl combine the crab meat, shrimp and sea salt.

When the eggs begin to bubble spread the seafood mixture over the top.

Cook 5 minutes or until the filling is hot.

Fold over in the middle and enjoy.

Shrimp Tomatoes

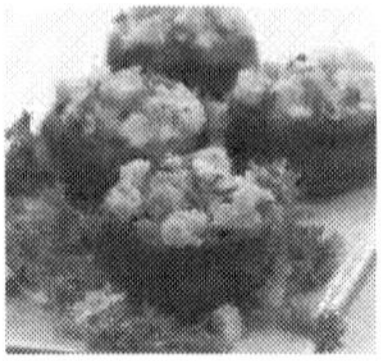

Ingredients:

3.5 oz. shrimp, cooked

Juice from 1 lemon

1 tbsp parsley

1/8 tsp salt

1/4 tsp pepper

2 tomatoes

1 dash of Tabasco sauce

Directions:

Pulse the shrimp in a food processor blender just enough to coarsely chop.

Place the chopped shrimp into a bowl and sprinkle with the lemon juice.

Stir in the parsley, salt and pepper.

Remove the tops and the pulp from the tomatoes and remove the seeds if you wish.

Chop the tomato pulp and place into the bowl with the shrimp, stirring to combine well.

Stuff the tomatoes with the shrimp mixture and add a dash of Tabasco sauce to each one.

Lightly Seasoned Crab Patties

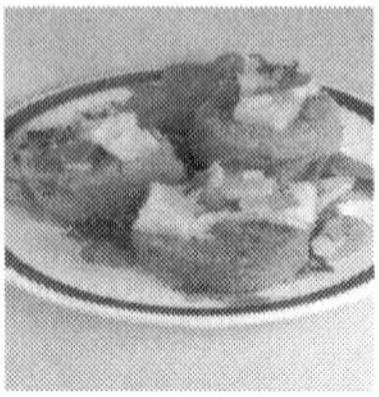

Ingredients:

1 grissini, ground very fine

3.5 oz. of crab meat

1 tsp parsley

1/2 tsp tarragon

1/2 tsp paprika

1/4 tsp white pepper

1/4 tsp cayenne pepper

1/4 tsp dry mustard

1/2 tsp lemon juice

Directions:

Put the grissini into a mixing bowl.

Place the crab and all the seasonings into a separate bowl.

Stir in the lemon juice and form the mixture into patties.

Coat the patties with the grissini powder on both sides.

Lay the patties into a skillet placed over medium heat.

Cook the crab patties for 3 minutes then flip.

Cook an additional 3 minutes or until lightly browned.

Grissini are thin dry bread sticks that can be found in most supermarkets. If you are having trouble finding grissini, Melba toast rounds will work just as well.

Cayenne Chili Shrimp

Cayenne Chili Shrimp

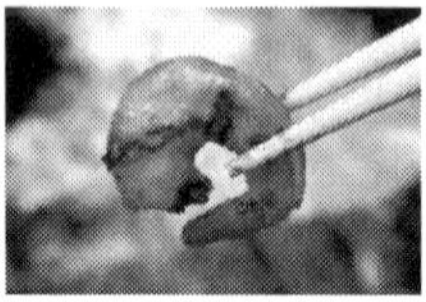

Ingredients:

3.5 oz. of precooked shrimp

1 tbsp chili powder

1 tbsp paprika

1 tsp onion powder

1 tsp garlic powder

1/2 tsp cayenne pepper

1/2 tsp oregano

1/2 tsp thyme

2 packets of Stevia sweetener

Directions:

Preheat an indoor grill.

Place the shrimp into a large bowl.

Mix together all of the seasonings and sweetener in a separate bowl until well blended.

Dip the shrimp into the seasoning coating them well.

Place on the preheated grill and cook for 4 minutes or until heated through.

If you are not fond of spicy shrimp you may omit the chili powder or the cayenne pepper or add a little less of each to the seasoning mixture.

Cajun Tilapia

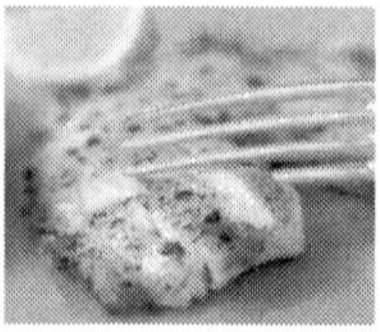

Ingredients:

2 tbsp extra virgin raw coconut oil

3.5 oz. of tilapia fillets

1/8 tsp paprika

1/8 tsp chili powder

1/8 tsp garlic salt

Directions:

Pour the oil into a skillet and place the skillet over medium heat.

Sprinkle the seasonings over both sides of the fillets.

Lay the fillets into the skillet and cook 3 minutes then turn.

Cook 2 minutes or until the internal temperature reaches 145 degrees.

Lemon Cod with Asparagus

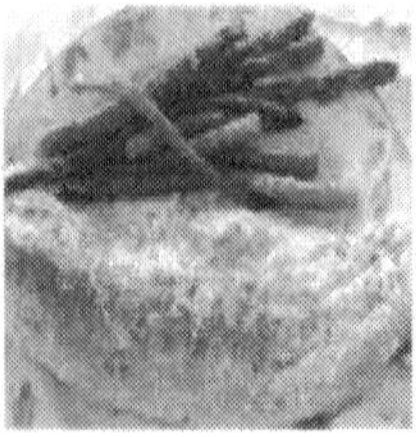

Ingredients:

3.5 oz. asparagus

3.5 oz. cod filets

1/4 tsp salt

1/4 tsp pepper

Juice from one fresh lemon

1 tbsp oregano

Directions:

Preheat the oven to 400 degrees and tear off a large sheet of aluminum foil.

Trim off the woody ends of the asparagus and place it in the middle of the foil.

Lay the cod fillets over the top of the asparagus and sprinkle with the salt and pepper.

Whisk the lemon juice and oregano together until well blended and pour over the fish.

Fold the foil over the food and seal tightly.

Bake for 15 minutes or until the fillets flake easily.

Lemon Pepper Halibut

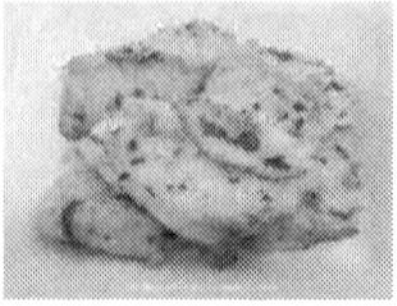

Ingredients:

2 garlic cloves, minced

1/2 tsp pepper

1/4 tsp turmeric

1/4 tsp cumin powder

1/4 tsp salt

Juice for a half of fresh lemon

3.5 oz. of halibut

Directions:

In a bowl whisk together the garlic, pepper, turmeric, cumin, salt and lemon juice.

Add the fish to the mixture, turning to coat, cover the bowl and refrigerate for 1 hour.

Set the oven temperature to 400 and preheat.

Place the marinated fish on a baking sheet and discard the marinade.

Bake for 18 minutes or until the fish flakes easily with a fork.

Seasoned Orange Chicken

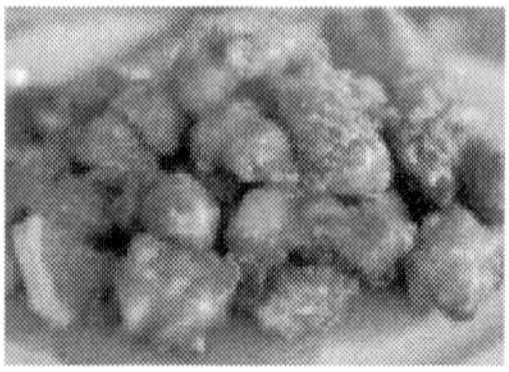

Ingredients:

3.5 oz. of chicken, cut into chunks

1/4 tsp of pepper

2 garlic cloves, minced

1 orange, peeled and cut into quarters

Juice from half of a lemon

1 tbsp fresh ginger root, peeled and minced

1/2 tsp of basil

Directions:

Preheat a skillet over medium heat.

Sprinkle the chicken with the pepper and place it in the hot skillet.

Stirring often, brown the chicken on all sides for 8 minutes or until completely browned.

Stir in the garlic and cook for 1 minute longer.

Squeeze the juice from the orange quarters over the chicken.

Separate the orange segments and gently stir them into the chicken.

Stir in the lemon juice, ginger and basil until well combined.

Cover the skillet and cook for 25 minutes or until the chicken is cooked through.

Broth Simmered Chicken

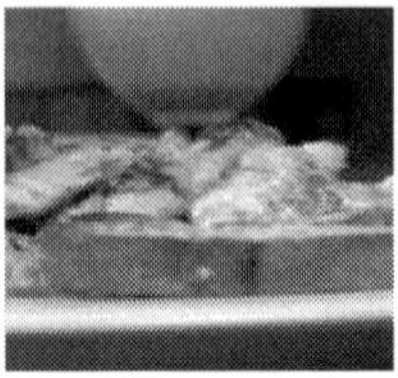

Ingredients:

3.5 oz. chicken breasts

1 tbsp oregano

2 tsp basil

1 C of homemade chicken broth

Juice from 1/2 of a lemon

3.5 oz. of tomatoes, chopped

1 tsp garlic salt

Directions:

Pound the chicken breasts flat using a meat mallet.

Sprinkle both sides the chicken evenly with the oregano and basil.

Place the flattened chicken into a saucepan.

Pour the broth over the chicken and squeeze in the lemon juice.

Stir in the tomatoes and garlic salt.

Cover and simmer over low heat for 1 hour or until the chicken is fork tender.

Remove the chicken from the broth and allow it to cool enough to handle.

Cut the chicken into strips and return to the broth before serving.

Parmesan Coated Chicken Tenders

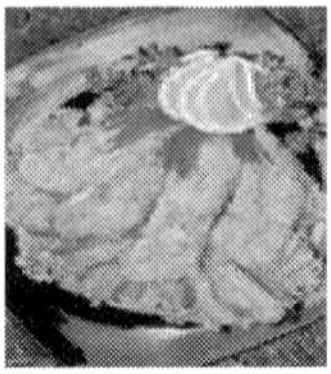

Ingredients:

1 C of egg whites

3.5 oz. chicken tenders

1/2 tsp salt

1/4 tsp pepper

1 1/4 C Parmesan cheese, grated

3/4 C Italian bread crumbs

Directions:

Place the egg whites into a small bowl and whisk slightly.

Sprinkle the chicken tenders with the salt and pepper.

Place the cheese and bread crumbs into a bowl and toss to combine.

Dredge the chicken tenders through the egg whites then through the crumbs coating well.

Place the oven on 475 degrees and preheat.

Spray a heavy oven proof skillet with cooking spray.

Place the tenders into the skillet and brown for 3 minutes per side.

Place the skillet into the oven and cook 10 minutes or until the chicken is cooked through.

Crock Pot Beef Roast

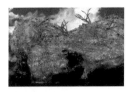

Ingredients:

1 (2 lb.) sirloin beef roast

1/2 C of water

3 tsp of garlic, minced

2 tbsp of oregano

1 tsp of salt

1 tsp of pepper

Directions:

Place the roast into the crock pot and pour the water over the top.

Spread the garlic over the top of the roast.

Sprinkle the roast with oregano, salt and pepper.

Cover the crock pot and cook on low for 12 hours or until the meat is cooked through.

Let the roast stand for 10 minutes before slicing or shredding.

Marinated Steak and Veggies

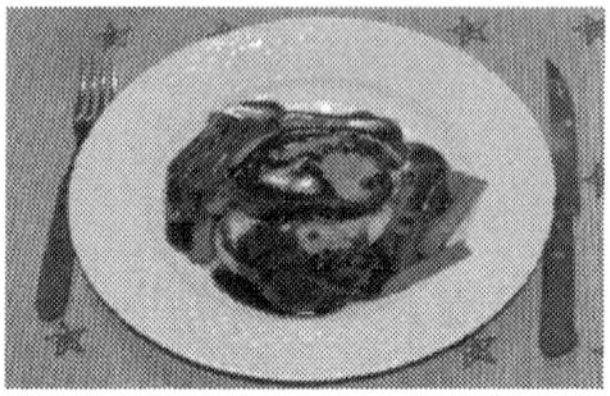

Ingredients:

1 tsp salt

1/2 tsp cumin

1/2 tsp onion powder

1/4 tsp garlic powder

1/4 C of water

3.5 oz. flat iron steak

1 bell pepper, cored, seed and cut into thin strips

1 onion, sliced thin

2 tbsp lime juice

Directions:

Place the salt, cumin, onion and garlic powder into a zip lock bag.

Add the water and shake to combine.

Place the steak, peppers, onion and lime juice into the bag and seal.

Turn the bag to coat the ingredients well.

Chill for at least 15 minutes

Heat a skillet over medium heat and add the marinated ingredients to the skillet.

Stirring often cook for 6 minutes, until the steak is cooked and the vegetables are tender.

Muffin Tin Meatballs

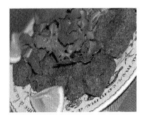

Ingredients:

19 oz. steak, ground

1 (8 oz.) can sugar free no salt tomato sauce

6 slices of Melba toast, ground fine

1 tbsp dried onions

1 egg

1 tsp salt

1/2 tsp pepper

Directions:

Allow the oven to preheat to 400 degrees.

Place the ground steak into a bowl.

Add the tomato sauce, ground toast crumbs, onions and egg.

Season the mixture with the salt and pepper.

Mix well to combine the ingredients.

Form the mixture into 18 meatballs that weigh 1.5 oz. each.

Lightly spray 2 mini muffin tins with cooking spray.

Place the meatballs into the prepared tins.

Bake the meatballs for 20 minutes or until completely cooked through.

Chili Spiced Beef Roast

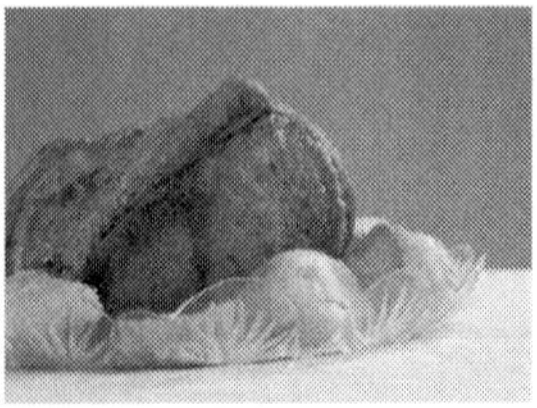

Ingredients:

1 (3 lb.) lean roast, all fat removed

6 garlic cloves

1 tsp salt

1/2 tsp garlic powder

1/2 tsp onion powder

1/2 tsp chili powder

1/4 tsp cayenne pepper

1/4 tsp black pepper

1 onion, cut into chunks

Directions:

Set the oven temperature to 350 degrees and let the oven preheat.

Place the roast into a roasting pan and add 1 inch of water to the pan.

Cut 6 slits into the top of the roast and place a garlic clove into each of the slits.

Mix together the salt, garlic, onion and chili powder and both types of pepper.

Rub the mixture over the roast.

Place the chunks of onion around the roast.

Place the roast in the oven and cook for 1 hour or until the roast is cooked through.

Garlic Roasted Asparagus

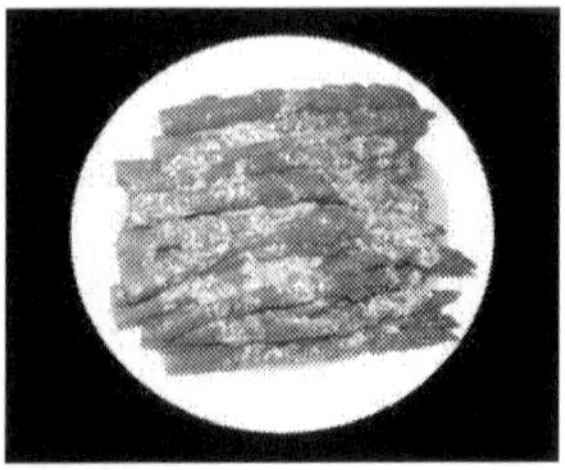

Ingredients:

3.5 oz. of asparagus

1 garlic clove, minced

1/2 tsp parsley

1/4 tsp oregano

1/8 tsp pepper

Directions:

Preset the oven temperature to 400 degrees allowing the oven to preheat.

Cover a baking sheet with aluminum foil.

Wash the asparagus and trim off any woody ends.

Place the asparagus in a single layer on the baking sheet.

Sprinkle the parsley, oregano and pepper over asparagus, turning to coat both sides.

Enclose the asparagus in the foil to seal it in.

Place in the oven and roast for 18 minutes or until tender.

Spicy Sweet Cucumber Slices

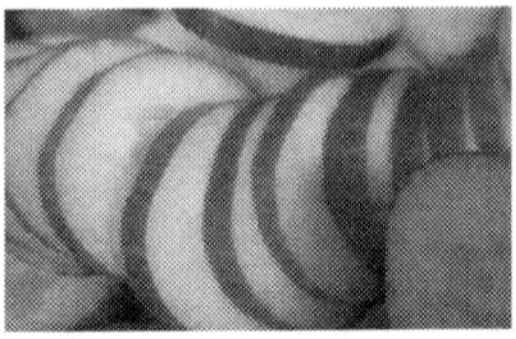

Ingredients:

1 large cucumber

1/8 tsp Cajun seasoning

1 packet of Stevia sweetener

Directions:

Peel the cucumbers if you wish then cut them into thin slices.

Place the cucumbers in an even layer onto a plate.

Sprinkle the Cajun seasoning and Stevia evenly over the top turning to coat well.

Oven Baked Onions

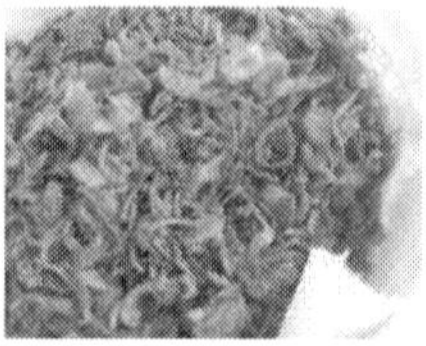

Ingredients:

1 tbsp skim milk

1/4 tsp cayenne pepper

1/4 tsp salt

1/4 tsp black pepper

1 Grissini breadstick

1 sweet onion, cut into very thin slices

Directions:

Set the oven temperature to 450 degrees and allow the oven to preheat.

Line a baking sheet with aluminum foil.

Whisk together the milk, cayenne pepper, salt and black pepper until well blended.

Place the grissini into the food processor and grind until it turns into a fine powder.

Coat the onions with the milk mixture being sure they are coated well.

Let the onions set in the batter for 2 minutes before removing.

Place the coated onions into the grissini powder, one at a time and roll to coat.

Place the onions onto the prepared baking sheet.

Bake for 6 minutes then flip and continue baking for an additional 6 minutes.

Lemon Cabbage

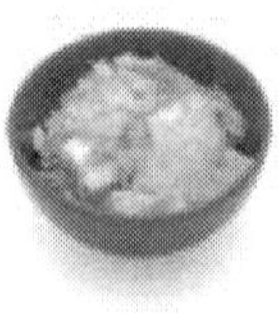

Ingredients:

1 head of cabbage, washed and drained well

Juice from one lemon

Salt to taste

Directions:

Place the cabbage in a steamer and steam for 10 minutes or until tender but not mushy.

Remove the cabbage and place it in a bowl.

Add the lemon juice to the cabbage and toss to coat.

Sprinkle with the salt to taste.

Herbed Mashed Cauliflower

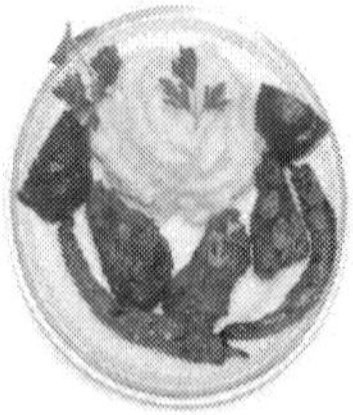

Ingredients:

1/4 C of water

1 (10 oz.) bag of frozen cauliflower

Herb seasoning salt to taste

Directions:

Pour the water into a saucepan and add the cauliflower.

Cook the cauliflower according to the package directions being sure it is quite soft.

Drain the cauliflower well and transfer to the blender.

Puree until smooth and creamy.

Season the cauliflower with the herb seasoning salt. .

Cinnamon Baked Apple Bites

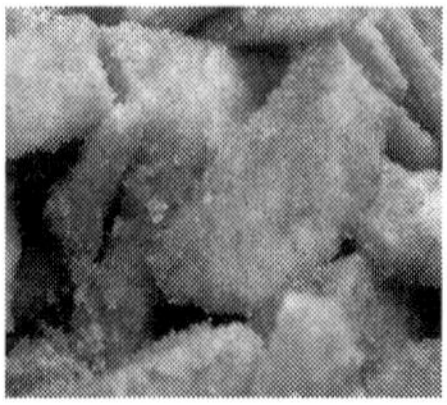

Ingredients:

3.5 oz. of Melba toast crumbs

1/2 tsp powdered Stevia

1/4 tsp of cinnamon

1/8 tsp of nutmeg

1/8 tsp of vanilla powder

1 apple, cored, peeled and cut into quarters

1 tsp of lemon juice

Directions:

Place the Melba toast crumbs into a mixing bowl.

Whisk in the Stevia, cinnamon, nutmeg and vanilla powder.

Place the apples in a separate bowl and sprinkle with the lemon juice.

Coat the apples with the Melba toast crumb mixture.

Place the coated apples on a baking sheet.

Bake the apples in a preheated 375 degree oven for 18 minutes or until soft.

Homemade Spiced Applesauce

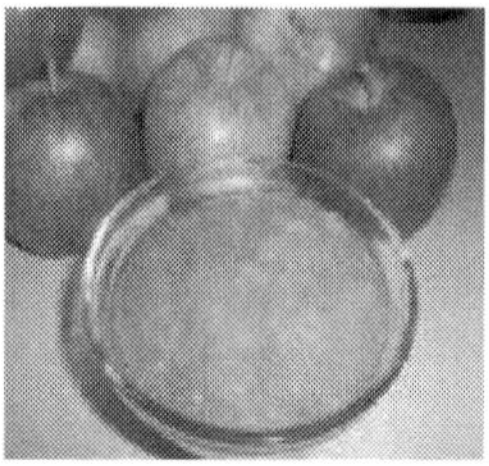

Ingredients:

1 sweet apple, peeled, cored and diced

3 tbsp of water

1 tsp of cinnamon

Directions:

Place the apples in a mini slow cooker.

Add the water and the cinnamon.

Cover the crock pot and cook on low for 3 hours or until the apples are very soft.

Transfer to the blender and blend until the desired consistency is reached.

Serve warm or refrigerate until ready to eat.

Broiled Caramelized Grapefruit

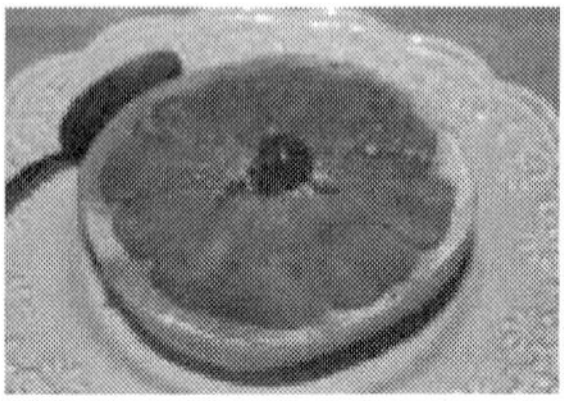

Ingredients:

1/2 of a grapefruit

1/8 tsp cinnamon

1/8 tsp of Stevia

Directions:

Place the oven on broil and preheat.

Separate the sections and place in an oven proof bowl.

If the grapefruit isn't producing a lot of juice add a little water to moisten.

Toss the cinnamon and Stevia together in a small bowl.

Sprinkle the mixture evenly over the grapefruit.

Place the bowl on a broiler pan and broil 6 inches from the heat.

Broil 3 minutes or until the top of the grapefruit has caramelized.

Cantaloupe Mix Fruit Bowl

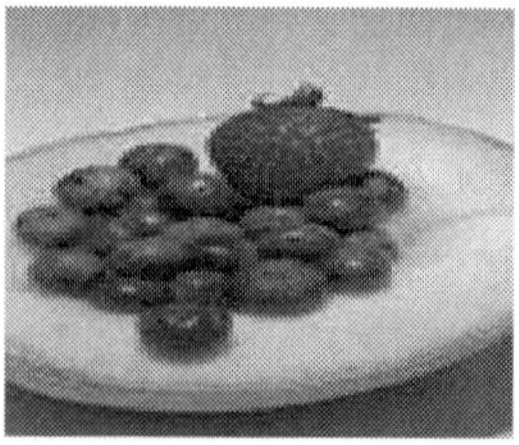

Ingredients:

1/2 cantaloupe

1/4 C of blueberries

1/4 C of strawberries, sliced

1 packet of Stevia sweetener

Directions:

Remove the seeds and membrane from the middle of the cantaloupe.

In a mixing bowl toss together gently the blueberries and strawberries.

Fill the center of the cantaloupe with the fruit mixture.

Sprinkle the Stevia over the top and enjoy.

Broccoli Pimiento Pasta

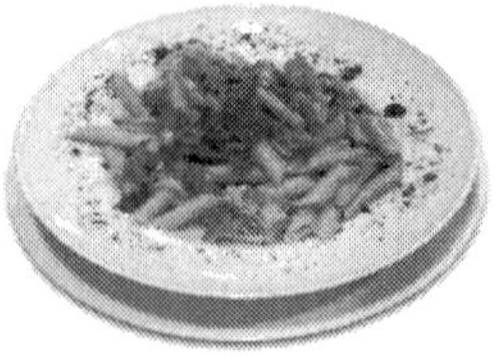

Ingredients:

1 (8 oz.) box of Ditalini pasta

2 tbsp of vegetable oil

1/2 tsp red pepper flakes

1 lb. broccoli florets

1/2 C of water

1 (6 oz.) jar of pimientos, drained

1 (6 oz.) jar of roasted peppers, drained and diced

1/4 C of Parmesan cheese, grated

Directions:

Cook the pasta as directed on the package, drain and set aside.

Pour the oil into a skillet and heat over medium heat.

Stir in the red pepper flakes and cook, stirring almost constantly for 2 minutes.

Stir in the broccoli and cook for 3 minutes.

Pour the water into the skillet, cover and steam for 3 minutes or until just tender.

Transfer the broccoli to the pasta,

Add the pimentos and peppers to the pasta and gently stir to combine.

Sprinkle with the Parmesan cheese just before serving.

Ditalini pasta is small tubular pasta that can be found in most grocery stores or supermarkets. If you can't find ditalini pasta any approved small tubular pasta will work.

Dilly Cucumber Salad

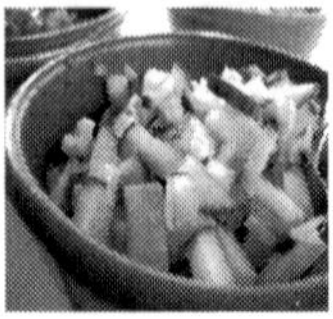

Ingredients:

3.5 oz. cucumbers, chopped

1 Tbsp vinegar

1 tsp dill

1/4 tsp Stevia

1/8 tsp pepper

Directions:

Place the chopped cucumbers into a salad bowl.

Whisk together the vinegar, dill, Stevia and pepper until well blended.

Pour over the cucumbers and toss to coat well.

Cover and refrigerate at least 30 minutes before serving.

Apple Celery Chicken Salad

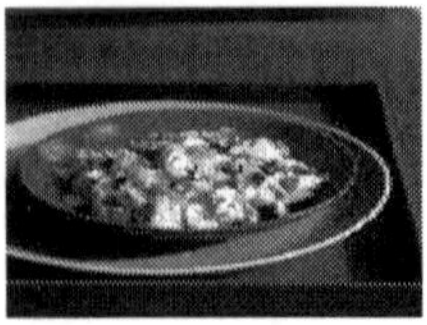

Ingredients:

3.5 oz. chicken, cooked and diced

1 sweet apple, cored and diced

2 celery stalks, diced

3 tbsp of lemon juice

1 dash of nutmeg

1 dash of cardamom

1/8 tsp cinnamon

1/8 tsp of Stevia

Directions:

Toss together the chicken, apple and celery.

Whisk together the lemon juice, nutmeg and cardamom.

Pour the dressing over the salad and toss to coat well.

Cover and chill for at least 20 minutes.

Just before serving, stir again and sprinkle with the cinnamon and Stevia.

Chicken Broth from Your Kitchen

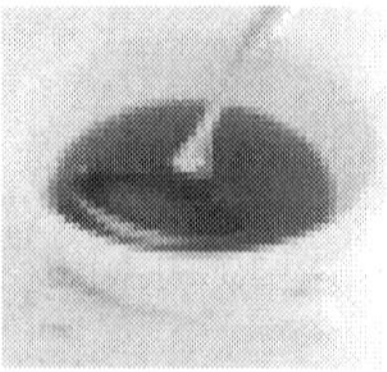

Ingredients:

6 (3.5 oz.) pieces of chicken breast

8 C of water

1/2 tsp sea salt

1/4 tsp garlic powder

1/4 tsp onion salt

1/4 tsp celery salt

1/4 tsp poultry seasoning

1/4 tsp pepper

Directions:

Place the chicken into a large soup pot.

Pour the water into the pot and place the pot over high heat.

Stir in all the seasonings and bring the water to a brisk boil.

Reduce the heat to medium low and cover the pot.

Simmer for 2 hours or until the chicken is cooked through.

Remove the chicken for later use.

Cool the broth before using.

This recipe makes 6 servings of chicken broth. Freeze it in containers for later use. It will stay fresh in the freezer for up to 2 months.

Chicken and Cabbage Chili

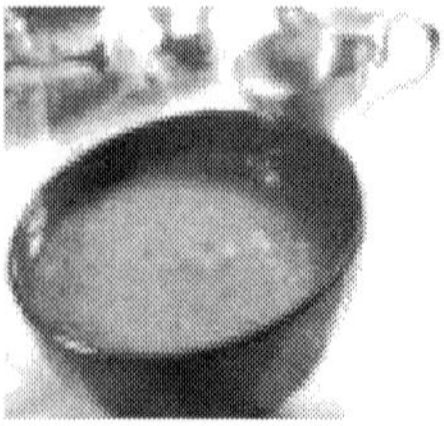

Ingredients:

2 C of homemade chicken broth

1 tbsp cumin

1 tbsp chili powder

1 tsp cayenne pepper

1 tsp black pepper

3.5 oz. cooked chicken, cubed

1 C of shredded cabbage

Directions:

Pour the broth into a saucepan and place over high heat.

Stir in the cumin, chili powder, cayenne and black pepper.

Bring the mixture to a boil.

Once boiling carefully stir in the chicken and cabbage.

Reduce the heat to medium and cover the pan.

Simmer the chili for 15 minutes or until heated through.

Roasted Garlic Tomato Soup

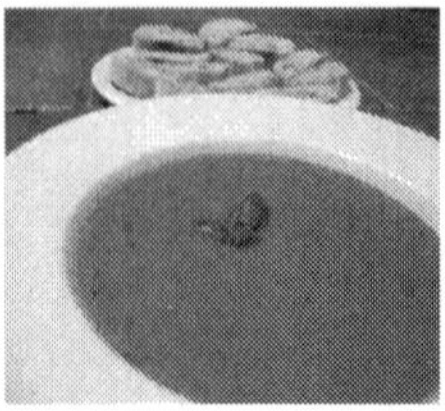

Ingredients:

2 large tomatoes, peeled and seeds removed

Homemade chicken broth

1 tbsp roasted garlic

1/2 tsp pepper

1/4 tsp salt

1 tbsp fat free milk

Directions:

Preset the oven to broil allowing it to preheat.

Place the tomatoes onto a broiler pan.

Broil the tomatoes for 6 minutes, watching them carefully so they don’t burn.

Remove the tomatoes and place them in a saucepan.

Pour enough chicken broth into the pan to completely cover the tomatoes.

Place the pan over high heat.

When the soup just begins to boil add in the roasted garlic.

Bring the soup to a full boil.

Pour the soup into the blender and sprinkle with the salt and pepper.

Add in the milk and blend until smooth.

Chicken and Spinach Soup

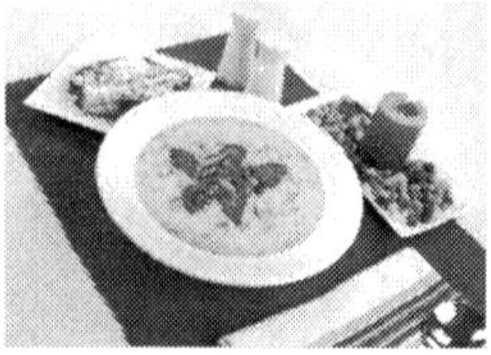

Ingredients:

3 C of homemade chicken broth

3.5 oz. cooked chicken breast, shredded

3.5 oz. fresh spinach

Juice from 1 lemon

1 tsp thyme

1/2 tsp salt

1/2 tsp white pepper

Directions:

Pour the broth into a large saucepan.

Add in the chicken and spinach.

Stir in the lemon juice, thyme, salt, and pepper.

Place the pan over high heat and bring to a boil.

Once boiling, reduce the heat to medium and simmer the soup for 20 minutes.

Autumn Chicken Soup

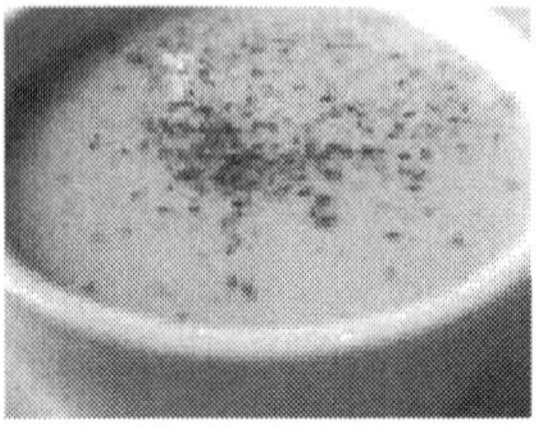

Ingredients:

3.5 oz. chicken, cubed

2 C of homemade chicken broth

3 garlic cloves, minced

1/2 tsp curry powder

1/4 tsp cinnamon

1/4 tsp pumpkin pie spice

1/4 tsp salt

1/4 tsp pepper

Directions:

Place the chicken into a saucepan placed over medium heat.

Pour the broth over the chicken and stir in the garlic.

Add the seasonings and stir to blend in.

Bring the soup to a rolling boil then reduce the heat to medium low.

Cover the pan and simmer 45 minutes.

Italian Vegetable Soup

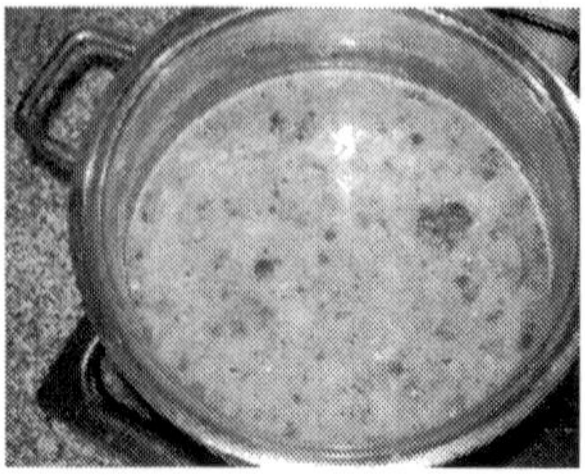

Ingredients:

8 C of homemade chicken broth

1 (29 oz.) can of crushed tomatoes, drained

1 onion, chopped

1/2 head of cabbage, torn

1/2 C of celery, sliced

1 tsp Italian seasoning

1/2 tsp pepper

Directions:

Pour the broth into a large soup pan and place the pan over high heat.

Stir in the tomatoes, onion, cabbage and celery.

Season the soup with the Italian seasoning and pepper stirring to blend in well.

Bring the soup to a boil then reduce the heat to medium low.

Simmer for 20 minutes or until the vegetables are as tender as you like.

No Cook Celery Soup

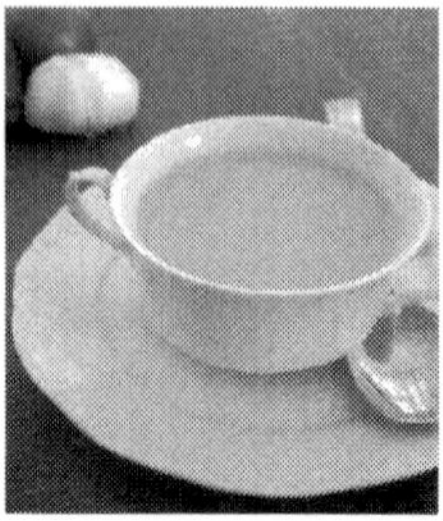

Ingredients:

1 C of water

1 1/2 scoops of protein powder

1 tsp minced onion

1 tsp garlic powder

1/2 tsp basil

1/4 tsp coriander

1/4 tsp pepper

1/8 tsp sea salt

3.5 oz. of celery, chopped fine

1 1/2 t Konjac flour

Directions:

Pour the water into the blender.

Add the protein powder, onion, garlic, basil, coriander, pepper and salt.

Gently add in the celery.

Puree for 1 minute or until smooth.

Add the flour and puree for an additional 1 minute to thicken.

Pour into a bowl and stir.

This soup can be heated in the microwave or on the stove if you wish. It may also be chilled if you like a nice refreshing chilled soup.

Apple Cider Shrimp Wraps

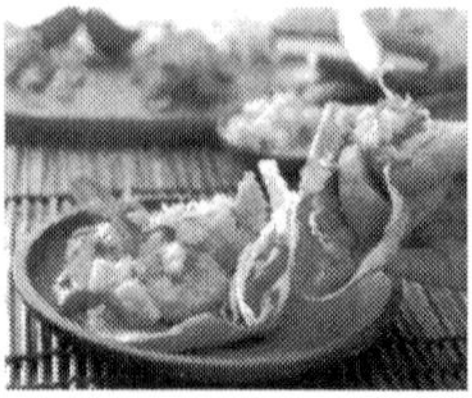

Ingredients:

3.5 oz. shrimp

1 tsp salt

2 Boston lettuce leaves

3 tbsp apple cider vinegar

1 garlic clove

1 tbsp fresh ginger

2 tsp garlic powder

Stevia to taste

Directions:

Place the shrimp into a saucepan and cover with water.

Sprinkle in the salt and place the pan over high heat.

Bring the water to a boil, reduce the heat to medium.

Simmer the shrimp for 5 minutes or until opaque in color.

Drain well and allow the shrimp to cool to room temperature.

Stir together the vinegar, clove, ginger and garlic powder until well blended.

Add Stevia to taste stirring to combine well.

Place the shrimp into the dressing mixture and turn to coat.

Add the shrimp to the lettuce leaves and wrap the leaves around the shrimp.

Pita Pepperoni Pizza

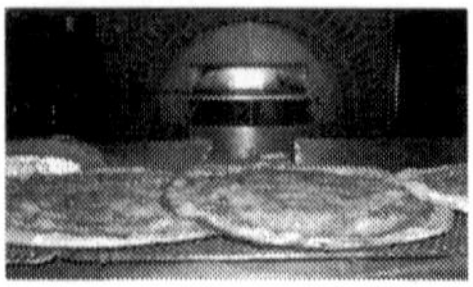

Ingredients:

1 piece of whole wheat pita bread

2 tbsp low sugar tomato sauce

1/4 tsp garlic, minced

1/2 tsp Italian seasoning

1/2 tsp Parmesan cheese

3.5 oz. sliced pepperoni

1/4 C mozzarella cheese, grated

Directions:

Set the oven to 425 degrees and preheat.

Place the pita onto a baking sheet and warm in the oven for 5 minutes.

Spread the tomato sauce evenly over the warmed pita.

In a mixing bowl toss together the garlic, Italian seasoning and Parmesan cheese.

Sprinkle the mixture evenly over the sauce.

Place the pepperoni over the pizza and top with the mozzarella cheese.

Bake 8 minutes or until the cheese has completely melted.

Melba Dutch Apple Pie

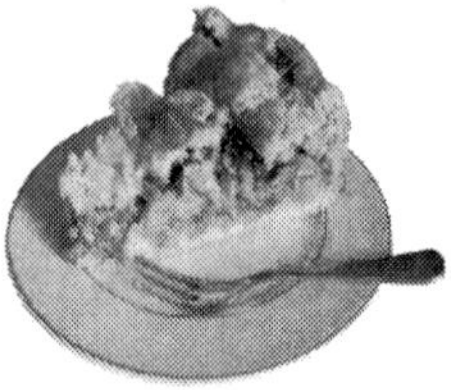

Ingredients:

2 pieces of Melba toast, crushed

2 pkg. Stevia sweetener, divided

1 1/2 tbsp cinnamon, divided

2 tbsp of water

1 large apple, cored, seed removed and sliced thin

Directions:

Place the crushed Melba toast into a mixing bowl.

Sprinkle in one pkg. of Stevia and 1/2 tsp of the cinnamon and mix well.

Divide the Melba toast mixture between 2 bowls.

Add the water to one bowl of the crust mix to moisten.

Press the mixture into the bottom of a soufflé dish.

Mix together the remaining Stevia and cinnamon.

Sprinkle the mixture over the apple slices and toss to coat.

Spread the apple slices over the bottom crust.

Cover the top with the remaining dry crumb mixture.

Bake the pie in a preheated 450 degree oven for 15 minutes or until nicely brown on top.

Layered Strawberry Pie

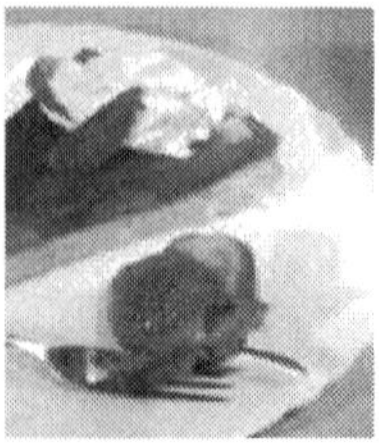

Ingredients:

6 oz. pecans, chopped

2 oz. walnuts, chopped

3 tbsp of butter, melted

2 tbsp Stevia sweetener

1 box sugar and fat free instant lemon pudding

1 C of cold milk

1 (8 oz.) pkg. fat free cream cheese

3 tbsp of lemon juice

1 C boiling water

3/4 C cold water

1 pkg. sugar free instant strawberry gelatin

1 C of strawberries, sliced

1/2 container of sugar free whipped topping

Directions:

Mix the nuts, butter and stevia together and press into the bottom and sides of a pie pan.

Bake in a preheated 350 degree oven for 10 minutes or until brown then cool.

Whisk together the pudding, milk, cream cheese and lemon juice and chill until set.

Spoon the mixture into the cooled pie crust.

Dissolve the gelatin in the boiling water then stir in the cold water.

Fold in the strawberries and chill until just beginning to set.

Fold in the whipped topping and spread the mixture over the top of the pie.

Chill until ready to serve.

Candy Bar Pudding

Candy Bar Pudding

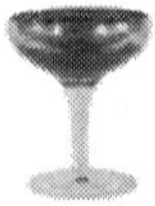

Ingredients:

32 g chocolate whey protein powder

1 1/2 tbsp all natural peanut butter

1/2 tsp unsweetened cocoa

1/8 tsp Stevia

2 tbsp water

Directions:

Place the whey powder, peanut butter and cocoa into a mixing bowl.

Sprinkle with the Stevia.

Whip the mixture adding a little water at a time until it reaches a pudding consistency.

Place into dessert glasses and enjoy.

Coconut Strawberry Pops

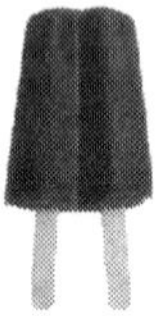

Ingredients:

1 scoop of protein powder

4 drops of strawberry flavored Stevia

1 can of coconut milk

Directions:

Pour the coconut milk into a mixing bowl.

Stir in the protein powder and Stevia.

Pour into Popsicle molds and freeze until solid.

Chocolate Strawberry Icee

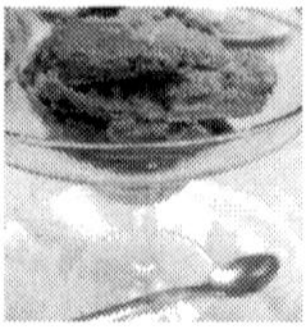

Ingredients:

3/4 C of water

1 1/2 scoops of natural flavored protein powder

5 drops of chocolate Stevia

4 frozen strawberries

7 ice cubes

Directions:

Pour the water into the blender.

Add in the protein powder and Stevia.

Place the strawberries into the blender.

Carefully add the ice cubes.

Blend the icee for 35 seconds or until mixed together well.

Natural Spinach Tortillas

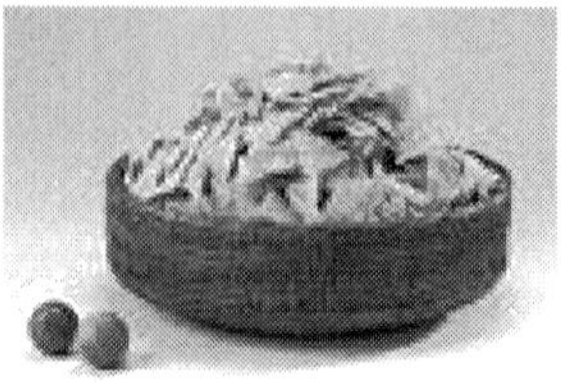

Ingredients:

1 lb. fresh spinach

Juice from one lemon

1 tsp salt

Directions:

Place the spinach onto mesh dehydrator sheets.

In a spritz bottle combine the lemon juice and salt.

Spritz the spinach thoroughly with the lemon salt mixture

Place in the dehydrator and dehydrate at 105 degrees until crunchy.

Homemade Shrimp Appetizer

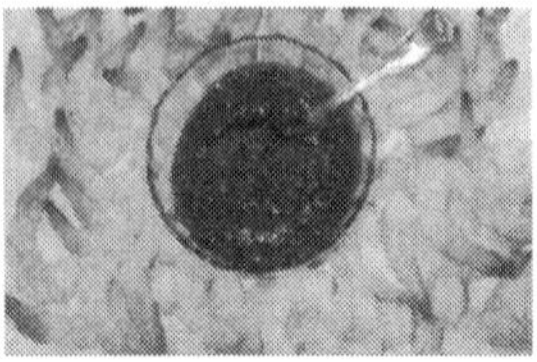

Ingredients:

1 (10 oz.) can organic, low sugar, low salt tomato sauce

2 tbsp onion powder

1 tbsp vinegar

1 tsp paprika

1 tsp horseradish

1/2 tsp sea salt

2 packets of Stevia

3.5 oz. of cold shrimp, washed, rinsed and deveined

Directions:

Dump the tomato sauce into a bowl.

Stir in the onion powder, vinegar, paprika and horseradish.

Add the sea salt and taste adding more if necessary.

Sprinkle in the Stevia and stir to blend in well.

Dip the shrimp into the cocktail sauce and enjoy.

Cherry Tomato Bruschetta

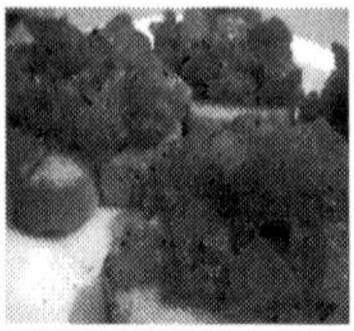

Ingredients:

1/2 C of cherry tomatoes, diced fine

1/4 C sweet onion, chopped fine

1/4 C fresh cilantro, chopped fine

2 tbsp balsamic vinegar

1 tsp salt

Melba toast

Directions:

Mix together the tomatoes, onions and cilantro.

Stir in the vinegar and salt and mix well.

Top the Melba toast with the Bruschetta.

Sparkling Strawberry Tea

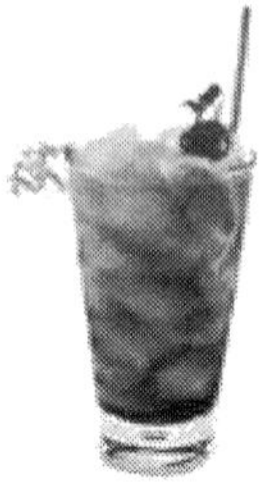

Ingredients:

4 fresh strawberries, washed and stems removed

1/2 C of brewed green tea, cold

1/2 C sparkling mineral water

2 T of lemon juice

Stevia to taste

Directions:

Place the strawberries into the food processor or blender and puree.

Pour the pureed berries through a fine mesh sieve to remove any seeds.

Place the puree into a bowl and stir in the tea and lemon juice.

Pour the mixture into a tall glass of ice.

Stir in the mineral water and Stevia well.

Chocolate Toffee Cappuccino

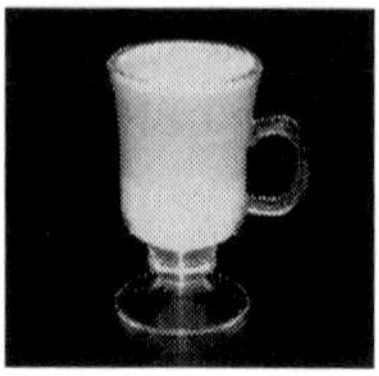

Ingredients:

1 C of coffee

5 drops of toffee flavored liquid Stevia

5 drops of chocolate flavored liquid Stevia

1 C of crushed ice

Directions:

Place the coffee and both of the flavored Stevia into the blender.

Add the crushed ice and blend until very smooth.

Spiced Up Apple Cider

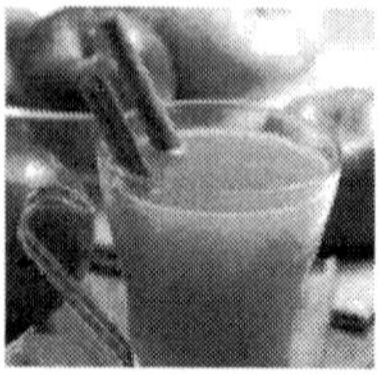

Ingredients:

The juice from 1 apple

2 tbsp lemon juice

1 tbsp apple cider vinegar

1/4 tsp cinnamon

1 dash of allspice

1 dash of nutmeg

1 dash of cloves

Stevia to taste

Directions:

Squeeze the apple juice into a saucepan and place the pan over medium heat.

Stir in the lemon juice and vinegar.

Sprinkle in the cinnamon, allspice, nutmeg and cloves.

If necessary you may add a little water to the mixture to have enough liquid for 1 serving.

Heat the mixture, stirring occasionally for 4 minutes or until heated through.

Strawberry Vanilla Smoothie

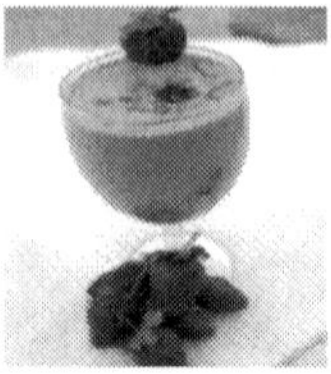

Ingredients:

1 C of frozen strawberries

1 pkg. Stevia sweetener

5 drops of orange Stevia

5 drops of vanilla cream Stevia

1 C of ice cubes

Directions:

Place the strawberries into a bowl.

Sprinkle the strawberries evenly with the Stevia tossing gently to coat.

Transfer the strawberries to the blender.

Add in the flavored Stevia and the ice cubes.

Blend until smooth and creamy.

Healthy Red Pop

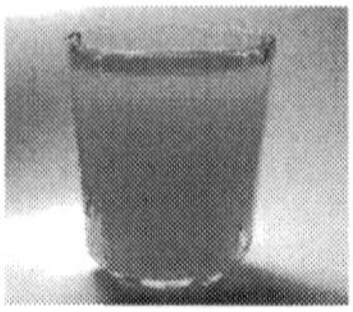

Ingredients:

6 strawberries

6 oz. club soda

Stevia to taste

Directions:

Place the strawberries into the blender.

Pour the club soda over the berries.

Cover and blend until smooth.

Pour into a glass of ice and add Stevia to taste.

Italian Meat Sauce

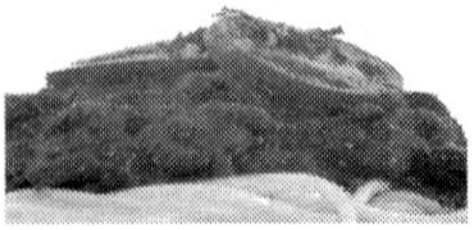

Ingredients:

1 large tomato cut into chunks

3.5 oz. lean ground beef

1/4 tsp garlic salt

1/4 tsp onion salt

1/4 tsp no carb Italian seasoning

Directions:

Place the tomatoes into a saucepan and place the pan over medium heat.

Cook the tomatoes, mashing them off and on to help soften them, for 8 minutes.

Cook the meat on an indoor grill for 7 minutes or until cooked through.

Crumble the cooked meat into the sauce and stir to combine.

Stir in the garlic salt, onion salt and Italian seasoning.

Cook the mixture, stirring often, for 10 minutes or until completely heated through.

9194376R0

Made in the USA
Lexington, KY
05 April 2011